I0074797

The Patient's Guide

Vascular Catheter Placement

Adam E. M. Eltorai, MD, PhD
Matthew Czar Taon, MD, RPVI, WCC
Terrance T. Healey, MD

Praeclarus Press, LLC
©2020 Matthew Czar Taon. All rights reserved.

www.PraeclarusPress.com

Praeclarus Press, LLC
2504 Sweetgum Lane
Amarillo, Texas 79124 USA
806-367-9950
www.PraeclarusPress.com

DISCLAIMER
The information contained in this publication is advisory only and
is not intended to replace sound clinical judgment or individualized
patient care. The author disclaims all warranties, whether expressed
or implied, including any warranty as the quality, accuracy, safety,
or suitability of this information for any particular purpose.

ISBN: 978-1-946665-30-0
©2020 Matthew Czar Taon. All rights reserved.
Email: matthew.taon@gmail.com

Cover Design: Ken Tackett
Developmental Editing: Kathleen Kendall-Tackett
Copy Editing: Chris Tackett
Layout & Design: Nelly Murariu

CONTENTS

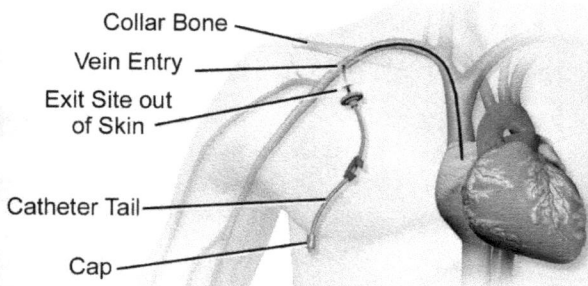

Collar Bone
Vein Entry
Exit Site out
of Skin

Catheter Tail
Cap

Non-Tunneled Central Venous Access Device

Central Venous Access Device (Non-Tunneled).

WHAT IS "VASCULAR CATHETER PLACEMENT?"

The term "**vascular**" refers to blood vessels and includes both arteries and veins. In general, arteries are blood vessels that provide oxygenated blood to tissues, while veins are blood vessels that transport deoxygenated blood (blood whose oxygen has been used and metabolized) from the tissues back to the heart.

A **catheter** is a thin, flexible, sterile plastic tube that can be placed into a blood vessel to facilitate blood draws for laboratory testing, medication administration, nutrition, blood transfusions, hemodialysis, or to provide hemodynamic or physiologic information about the patient's circulatory system.

There are different types of vascular catheters that can be placed depending on the clinical indication. One general method to organize the types of vascular catheters is to divide it into **venous** or **arterial** catheters. Venous catheters can be further subdivided into peripheral or central venous catheters. Regardless of the type of catheter being placed, placement follows similar principles. A needle is introduced into the vessel of interest and subsequently exchanged for a thin catheter. The catheter is then affixed to the patient's skin using an adhesive dressing, or in this case, central venous catheters with sutures.

A peripheral intravenous (IV) catheter is placed into a **peripheral vein** (arms, hands, legs, or feet) and is the most commonly utilized vascular catheter in medicine. Two types of peripheral intravenous catheters include short peripheral intravenous catheters and midline catheters. Short peripheral intravenous catheters measure less than 7.5 cm (3 inches) in length and are usually used for short-term venous access estimated to be less than 96 hours. Midline catheters measure 7.5 cm (3 inches) to 20 cm (8 inches) in length and are usually placed into a peripheral vein in the inner arm with catheter tip ending within a peripheral vein at the level of the shoulder or axilla. They are generally used for short-term or intermediate-term venous access estimated to range from 5 to 28 days.

A central venous catheter is a catheter that has a tip that ends within a **central vein** in the chest, abdomen, or pelvis. Central venous catheters can be placed through a peripheral vein, such as with a peripherally inserted central catheter (PICC) or a central vein, such as the internal jugular vein, subclavian vein, or femoral vein. Regardless of whether the venous access site is through a peripheral or central vein, the tip of a central venous catheter must end within a central vein.

Central venous catheters can be divided into 4 types: **peripherally inserted central catheters (PICC)**, temporary non-tunneled central venous catheters, permanent tunneled central venous catheters, and subcutaneous implanted port catheters. Peripherally inserted central catheters (PICC) are placed via a peripheral vein but extend within the venous system to end within a central vein. These are typically used for administration of intermediate-term medications such as antibiotics. **Non-tunneled central venous catheters** are generally used for short-term access to the central veins for treatments, which include vasoactive medications (medications that affect blood vessel size and diameter), emergent hemodialysis, intravenous nutrition known as total parenteral nutrition (TPN), or for obtaining pressures of the central veins. In patients who require central venous access for longer than 2 weeks, **tunneled central venous catheters** are the preferred catheter choice. **Port catheters** are composed of a reservoir hub, which is implanted beneath the skin of the arm or chest, and a catheter, which is tunneled beneath the skin to the accessed vein and extends within the vein to end within a central vein. Port catheters are used in patients who require long-term intermittent central venous access, such as with chemotherapy. When compared with each of the central venous catheter types, port catheters demonstrate the lowest incidence of infection since they are completely buried beneath the skin without exposure to the open environment.

Arterial catheters can be placed into the radial, brachial, axillary, or femoral arteries and are used primarily for direct intra-arterial blood pressure monitoring. Direct blood pressure monitoring differs from the blood pressure measurements obtained using a blood pressure cuff (sphygmomanometry), which is referred to as indirect blood pressure measurements. Indirect blood pressure measurement techniques often provide inaccurate blood pressure values since the measurements are not obtained directly within the artery. Inaccurate blood pressure measurements can have dire consequences in patients suffering from poor delivery of blood to their organs (circulatory shock), and may result in suboptimal disease management or death. In contradistinction, direct measurement of intraarterial blood pressure provides the most accurate blood pressure values since there is a catheter inside of the artery obtaining direct blood pressure measurements. Thus, direct intra-arterial blood pressure monitoring is preferred over indirect blood pressure monitoring in critically ill patients.

WHY IS VASCULAR CATHETER PLACEMENT PERFORMED?

Vascular catheters are performed for various clinical indications. Peripheral intravenous (IV) catheters are placed to facilitate blood draws for laboratory evaluation, fluid administration, medication administration, or intravenous contrast injection for radiologic imaging. Peripheral IV catheters are used for short-term venous access estimated to last less than 96 hours.

Midline catheter placement is indicated in patients who may require prolonged intravenous infusions, multiple laboratory draws, or who are known to have difficult peripheral venous access requiring multiple attempts. In general, midline catheters are used for short-term or intermediate-term venous access in the range between 5 to 28 days. The Centers for Disease Control (CDC) recommends that physicians consider placement of a midline catheter when the duration of intravenous therapy is predicted to exceed 6 days.

Peripherally inserted central catheters (PICCs) can be placed if there is a need for long-term intravenous (IV) antibiotics, intravenous nutrition (total parenteral nutrition), fluids, or other medications. PICCs may be preferred over other direct central venous access sites in patients with an increased bleeding risk due to low platelets, in patients with history of venous occlusions, or in obese patients in whom venous access may be difficult to obtain.

Non-tunneled central venous catheters are commonly placed

when there is an emergent need for large volume fluids, medications, or hemodialysis. In addition, vasoactive medications that cause changes in the diameter of the vessels are more appropriately administered via non-tunneled central venous catheters, rather than peripheral IVs. Compared to tunneled central venous catheters, non-tunneled central venous catheters are associated with a higher risk of infection and are preferred to remain in place for less than 2 weeks.

Tunneled central venous catheters are used in patients requiring long-term medication, fluid, nutrition, chemotherapy, or hemodialysis administration for a period greater than 2 weeks. Since the catheter is tunneled beneath the skin, it is more secure and has a lower associated risk of infection.

Port catheters are composed of a subcutaneous reservoir implanted within the chest wall or upper arm, which is connected to a tunneled catheter that resides within a central vein. These are primarily utilized in patients with cancer who are undergoing long term chemotherapy. Since port catheter are completely subcutaneous, they tend to have the least interference with a patient's daily activities and markedly reduced risk of infection compared to other central venous access options.

HOW DO I PREPARE FOR MY VASCULAR CATHETER PLACEMENT PROCEDURE?

Prior to placement of any vascular catheter, you should report to your doctor all medications that you are taking, including herbal supplements, and any allergies you may have, especially to local anesthetic medications, sedation medication, general anesthesia, or to contrast materials containing iodine (X-ray dye).

Depending on what type of vascular catheter is placed, your physician may advise you to stop taking aspirin, nonsteroidal anti-inflammatory drugs (NSAIDs), or blood thinners for a specified period of time before your procedure.

Women should inform their physician of any possibility that they may be pregnant in order to limit possible fetal radiation exposure.

Prior to the placement of a central venous catheter, you may undergo laboratory blood testing to assess kidney function and procedural bleeding risk. In addition, you may be instructed to avoid consuming food or drink for several hours before your procedure. Since sedation medication may be used during the procedure, you should plan to have a relative or friend drive you home afterward.

You may be asked to remove clothing, jewelry, dental appliances, and eyeglasses during the exam and may be requested to change into a gown.

Some vascular catheters may need to be placed when a patient is critically ill. In these cases, a spouse or **designated person of authority (DPOA)** may be requested to sign consent for a vascular catheter placement procedure.

WHAT IS THE EQUIPMENT LIKE?

Equipment used for vascular catheter placement may include fluoroscopy (live X-ray), ultrasound, a light-based vein finder, a needle, a guidewire, and a vascular access catheter.

Fluoroscopy is a live X-ray used to provide real-time imaging of vascular catheter placement. Ultrasound uses sound waves to provide real-time imaging of vascular catheter placement. A light-based vein finder may use light-emitting diodes (LED) or near-infrared light to highlight and map the location of peripheral veins for access.

The needles used to obtain peripheral IV access range in diameter from 0.7 mm (24 **Gauge**) to 1.9 mm (14 Gauge) and range in length from 1.5 cm to 3 cm. Central venous catheters range in diameter from 0.2 cm (6 **French**) to 0.43 cm (13 French) and range in length from 15 cm to 30 cm. Peripherally inserted central catheters (PICCs) range in diameter from 0.13 cm (4 French) to 0.23 cm (7 French) and are among the longest catheters ranging in length from 50 to 70 cm. Port catheters are composed of a subcutaneous reservoir hub and tunneled venous catheter. The reservoir hub comes in various shapes, approximately the diameter of a quarter, and is buried subcutaneously within the chest wall or upper arm.

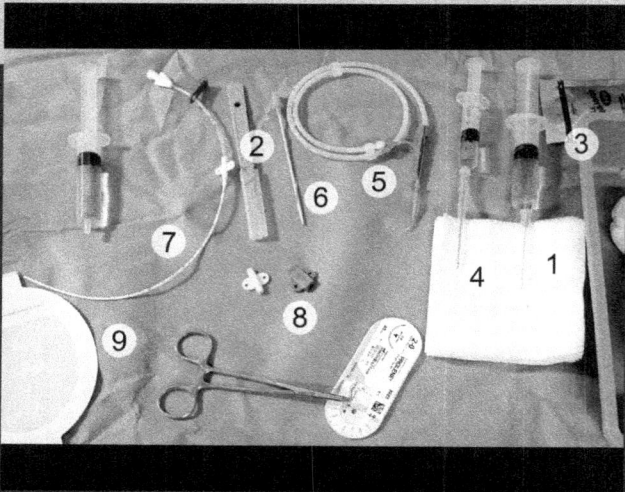

Central line equipment, in order of typical usage: Syringe with local anesthetic Scalpel in case venous cutdown is needed Sterile gel for ultrasound guidance Introducer needle (here 18 Ga) on syringe with saline to detect backflow of blood upon vein penetration Guide wire Tissue dilator Indwelling catheter (here 16 Ga) Additional fasteners, and corresponding surgical thread Dressing

WHAT DOES THE PROCEDURE INVOLVE?

Peripheral IV: Using a tourniquet, manual palpation, a light-based vein finder, or an ultrasound machine, a nurse will identify a peripheral vein, access it using a catheter-over-needle device, confirm adequate blood withdrawal, and affix the peripheral IV to the skin.

Peripherally-inserted central venous catheter (PICC): Using real-time ultrasound guidance, a physician or specially trained nurse will identify the basilic, cephalic, or brachial vein in the arm, access it using a needle and wire, replace the needle with a catheter, and advance the catheter until it is in the appropriate position within a central vein. A small amount of blood will be aspirated and flushed back into the catheter to ensure the functionality of the PICC. Then, the PICC will be sutured and affixed to the skin.

Non-tunneled central venous catheter: A physician will identify the internal jugular vein, subclavian vein, or femoral vein using manual palpation, anatomic landmarks, or real-time ultrasound guidance. After administering local anesthesia, the physician will use a needle and wire to access the vein and subsequently exchange the needle for a catheter directly into a central vein. After ensuring appropriate functionality, the non-tunneled central venous catheter will then be sutured and affixed to the skin.

Tunneled central venous catheter: A physician will identify the internal jugular vein, subclavian vein, or femoral vein using manual palpation, anatomic landmarks, or real-time ultrasound guidance. After administering sedation medication and local anesthesia, a physician will use a needle and wire to access the vein. The needle will be exchanged for a sheath to maintain access to the vein while minimizing the risk of injuring adjacent tissue. Subsequently, the physician will create a short, subcutaneous tunnel beneath the skin adjacent to the initial venous access site. A catheter will be advanced through the subcutaneous tunnel and into the venous access site. After ensuring appropriate functionality, the tunneled central venous catheter will be sutured and affixed to the skin.

Implanted port catheter: A physician will identify the internal jugular vein or subclavian vein using manual palpation, anatomic landmarks, or real-time ultrasound guidance. After administering sedation medication and local anesthesia, a physician will use a needle and wire to access the vein. The needle will be exchanged for a sheath to maintain access to the vein while minimizing the risk of injuring adjacent tissue. Subsequently, the physician will create a small subcutaneous pocket and short, subcutaneous tunnel beneath the skin adjacent to the initial venous access site. A port catheter will be advanced through the subcutaneous tunnel and into the venous access site while leaving the port reservoir hub nestled within the subcutaneous pocket. The skin incisions will then be sutured closed, thereby ensuring the entire port catheter system is closed to the environment.

Arterial catheter: A physician will identify the radial artery, brachial artery, axillary artery, or femoral artery using manual palpation, anatomic landmarks, or real-time ultrasound guidance. After administering local anesthesia, the physician will use a needle and wire to access the artery and subsequently exchange the needle for a catheter directly into the artery. After ensuring appropriate functionality, the arterial catheter will be sutured and affixed to the skin.

WHAT DOES VASCULAR CATHETER PLACEMENT FEEL LIKE?

When placing a peripheral IV, patients may experience a pinching and burning sensation while venous access is being obtained. This discomfort can be minimized with the use of topical anesthetic creams. Once the peripheral IV catheter is in place, there is minimal discomfort remaining.

When placing a non-tunneled central venous catheter, PICC, or arterial catheter, patients may experience a pinching and burning sensation due to the use of local anesthesia. Once effective local anesthesia is administered, patients may feel pressure during the procedure, but the sensation of pain should be minimized. Once the non-tunneled central venous catheter, PICC, or arterial catheter is in place, patients will have the catheter's external tubing affixed to their skin for the duration that the catheter is clinically indicated.

When placing a tunneled central venous catheter or port catheter, sedation medication, and local anesthesia may be utilized. Sedation medication functions to reduce anxiety, pain, and depress consciousness. Patients may feel drowsy due to sedation medications but are expected to retain the capacity to respond to tactile or verbal stimuli and maintain respiratory function. Once a tunneled central venous catheter is in place, patients will have the catheter's external tubing affixed to their skin for the duration that the catheter is clinically indicated. Alternatively, once an implanted port catheter is in place, patients will have a palpable port reservoir hub in their chest or upper arm but will not have external catheter tubing present.

WHAT HAPPENS AFTER THE PROCEDURE?

After a vascular catheter is placed, it is usually ready for immediate use. Patients will be able to receive their clinically indicated treatments immediately. Once the catheter is no longer indicated, it can be removed safely. In the setting of peripheral IVs, PICCs, and non-tunneled central venous catheters, once the catheter is removed, hemostasis is usually obtained by applying manual pressure. In the setting of tunneled central venous catheters and implanted port catheters, patients must return to the department, which placed the catheter for safe removal of the device. If you have questions during or after the procedure, you may be able to have them answered right then and there. Let your physician know your concerns, and he or she may be able to discuss them with you during or after the procedure.

How will I know the results of my procedure?

Once a vascular catheter is placed, it is usually ready for immediate use. Before the procedure officially ends, the catheter is tested to make sure it functions appropriately. Thus, you will know immediately whether the vascular catheter placement was successful.

WHAT ARE THE RISKS OF VASCULAR CATHETER PLACEMENT? WHAT ARE THE BENEFITS?

Risks of vascular catheter placement include non-infectious and infectious complications.

Noninfectious complications include:

⚠ damage to the blood vessel (vascular perforation),

⚠ bruising,

⚠ bleeding at the puncture site,

⚠ incorrect catheter placement,

⚠ damage to adjacent tissues,

⚠ injury to the lung or pleural lining of the lung causing gas to accumulate between the lung and chest wall (pneumothorax),

⚠ air embolism into the blood vessel,

⚠ arrhythmia,

⚠ blood clots,

⚠ catheter occlusion,

⚠ catheter dislodgement,

⚠ direct injury to the heart,

⚠ injury to the tissue surrounding the heart causing abnormal accumulation of fluid (pericardial effusion or cardiac tamponade).

Although rare, any of these potential complications, if severe enough, may result in death.

Infections associated with catheters can range in severity and include:

⚠ superficial skin infections near the access site,

⚠ catheter-related bloodstream infections,

⚠ sepsis (a disease process that results in poor blood perfusion throughout the body, multiorgan failure, and possible death).

Benefits of vascular catheter placement include:

- ✓ high volume,

- ✓ rapid fluid administration,

- ✓ lab draw accessibility,

- ✓ intravenous nutrition (total parenteral nutrition),

- ✓ blood product transfusion,

- ✓ medication administration,

- ✓ hemodialysis,

- ✓ chemotherapy administration,

- ✓ intravenous contrast administration,

- ✓ hemodynamic monitoring.

Risks and benefits of any procedure must be weighed carefully with the patient's current clinical scenario. It is prudent to frequently assess the need for all vascular catheters present and remove them as soon as safely possible.

Are there limitations to vascular catheter placement?

Vascular catheters can only provide value if they can be successfully placed within the appropriate vessel. Some patients may not have suitable blood vessels for vascular catheter placement due to prior injury, small caliber, or chronic occlusions. Other patients may not be suitable due to increased bleeding risk or abnormal anatomy.

In addition, vascular catheters are limited by the amount of time they can remain within the body. For example, peripheral IVs are recommended to be replaced within 96 hours. Alternatively, port catheters can remain in place for years but are often rated for a specific number of needle cannulations (i.e. 1000 versus 2000 needle cannulations).

FREQUENTLY ASKED QUESTIONS

Does vascular catheter placement involve any radiation?

It depends. Placement of a central venous catheter may require fluoroscopy (live X-rays), which involves radiation. Ultrasound imaging and light-based vein finders do not use radiation to identify blood vessels.

How long will my vascular catheter placement procedure take?

Peripheral IV placement can be performed in a matter of minutes. Central venous catheter and arterial catheter placement can take 30 minutes to an hour to perform.

When can my vascular catheter be removed?

It varies depending on the clinical scenario. Peripheral IVs can be removed the same day, whereas port catheters may remain in place for years.

What precautions are taken to limit catheter-related bloodstream infections?

There are 5 key measures that can reduce the incidence of catheter-related bloodstream infections: hand hygiene, procedural barrier precautions, skin antisepsis prior to catheter placement, appropriate cannulation site usage, and prompt catheter removal when it is no longer clinically indicated.

Does right- or left-handedness affect which arm a vascular catheter is placed?

In patients with renal disease who may require arteriovenous fistula placement in the future, right- or left-handed does play a role in which arm a vascular catheter is placed. Since fistulae are commonly placed in the nondominant arm, a PICC or subclavian central venous catheter should be inserted into the dominant arm.

GLOSSARY

VASCULAR

A term referring to blood vessels, namely arteries or veins.

CATHETER

A thin, flexible, sterile plastic tubing that can be placed into a blood vessel to facilitate blood draws for laboratory testing, medication administration, nutrition, blood transfusions, hemodialysis, or to provide hemodynamic or physiologic information about the patient's circulatory system.

PERIPHERAL VEIN

A smaller-caliber vein in the arms, hands, legs, or feet.

CENTRAL VEIN

A larger, vein located in the chest, abdomen, or pelvis (i.e., internal jugular vein, subclavian vein, superior vena cava, inferior vena cava, femoral vein).

PERIPHERALLY INSERTED CENTRAL CATHETER (PICC)

A catheter that is initially placed within a peripheral vein but extends within the venous system to end within a central vein.

NON-TUNNELED CENTRAL VENOUS CATHETER

A catheter that is not tunneled underneath the skin, used for short-term access to the central veins.

TUNNELED CENTRAL VENOUS CATHETER

A catheter tunneled beneath the skin used in patients who require central venous access for longer than 2 weeks.

PORT CATHETER

A device that consists of a reservoir hub, implanted beneath the skin of the arm or chest, and a tunneled catheter, used in patients who require long-term intermittent central venous access.

DESIGNATED PERSON OF AUTHORITY (DPOA)

A person designated with the authority to make healthcare decisions on behalf of another person.

GAUGE

A sizing system initially developed for iron wires but later adopted for hollow needles and catheters. Each gauge size is associated with a range of outer diameters. There is no fixed relationship between gauge size and actual mm size.

FRENCH

A vascular catheter sizing system in which 1 French is equal to 0.33 mm.

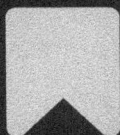

ADDITIONAL RESOURCES

Centers for Disease Control and Prevention:
Frequently Asked Questions about Catheters

https://www.cdc.gov/hai/bsi/catheter_faqs.html

American Thoracic Society Central Venous
Catheter Patient Education Series

https://www.thoracic.org/patients/patient-
resources/resources/central-venous-catheter.pdf

American Cancer Society:
Central Venous Catheters

https://www.cancer.org/treatment/treatments-
and-side-effects/central-venous-catheters.html

MY CONTACTS

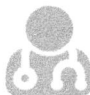

NAME

CONTACT

NAME

CONTACT

NAME

CONTACT

NAME

CONTACT

MY APPOINTMENTS

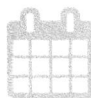

MONDAY

Date:
_____

THURSDAY

Date:
_____

TUESDAY

Date:
_____

FRIDAY

Date:
_____

WEDNESDAY

Date:
_____

SATURDAY

Date:
_____

MY QUESTIONS

MY QUESTIONS

MY QUESTIONS

MY QUESTIONS

MY QUESTIONS

MY NOTES

MY NOTES

MY NOTES

_____

_____

_____

_____

_____

_____

_____

_____

_____

_____

_____

MY NOTES

MY NOTES

MY NOTES

_____

_____

_____

_____

_____

_____

_____

_____

_____

_____

_____

_____

www.ingramcontent.com/pod-product-compliance
Lightning Source LLC
Chambersburg PA
CBHW071335200326
41520CB00013B/2995